Brianne Grebil

Love doesn't care if you forget

Lessons of Love from Alzheimer's and Dementia

To Mom and Dad, with all my heart

Contents

Praise for
Love Doesn't Care if You Forget

"The poet Robert Frost once wrote 'No tears in the writer, no tears in the reader.' This beautiful book is filled with tears – tears of sadness, tears of hope, tears of laughter, and above all tears of love. For anyone dealing with the slow and silent loss of a loved one to Alzheimer's and dementia, reading this short but powerful book will help you feel more peaceful and less alone than ever before."

Michael Neill, bestselling author of *The Inside-Out Revolution* and *The Space Within*

"What a beautiful book. I cried all the way through – it's perfect. So touching, so heartfelt. And a perfect length – so easily readable and simple in its message, whoever you are."

Nicola Bird, author of *A Little Peace of Mind*

Forward

If you have a Loved One who is experiencing dementia, this book will help you like no other. Brianne ever so clearly relates how she found beauty within the ordeal of Alzheimer's and dementia. As she journeyed with her mother, Brianne found joy in the pain and sublimity in the chaos. Reading these pages will plant seedlings of wisdom in your heart that will sprout one by one, just as you need them.

Brianne says: "When we focus on the disease, all we can see is what can be lost. We see all the things that are going wrong, all the things we cannot fix. And there we find despair, heartbreak, confusion, helplessness." For most of us, when we find ourselves traveling the dementia path with a Loved One, that is all we find.

But in these pages Brianne will show you how to go beyond the losses—to the great truths I have found myself, through dementia. As Brianne tells us: "Beyond all ideas, thought, feelings, words, language, Love itself is what carries us when we cannot carry ourselves."

But just a few words from me cannot relate the profound truth behind this simple statement. Read these pages and you'll find solace and discovery too.

Judy Cornish

Founder of the Dementia & Alzheimer's Wellbeing Network (DAWN)®
Author of *The Dementia Handbook* and *Dementia With Dignity*

Preface

"It is often in the darkest skies that we see the brightest stars."

Richard Evans

This small book is a message of deep Love and eternal hope. But the journey did not start there; far from it.

It started in fear and anguish on a cool afternoon in early October 2015. I sat with my father and mother in the neurologist's office. We listened as the doctor listed all the things that were *not* wrong with my mom.

"All her physical tests came back normal," he said and then rattled off all her normalcies. "Cardiology reports look good. Nutrient levels are normal. Blood pressure, blood sugar, blood count, all are fine."

What wasn't good in my mother's world? What wasn't normal or fine? Well, she'd forgotten how to tell time on a clock. She couldn't find the 4th of July on a calendar of July. She couldn't remember how many nieces and nephews she had, or even her own birthday.

Alzheimer's is a word that you never want to hear as a diagnosis, ever. Certainly not for someone at the relatively young age of 62. But that was the only word the doctor could offer us as an explanation. Early-onset Alzheimer's.

I was already familiar with this word. A few relatives on my mother's side had passed away with Alzheimer's and other dementias. But at the time I was young and they were old. They were my "great" relatives. My great-grandfather. My great-aunts. Someone in their 80s becoming feeble and demented just seemed like something that happened to older people in life. I was removed from it. What Alzheimer's meant to me growing up was distant. It was on the periphery of my life. It was never front and center. Until that day in the doctor's office with my mom and dad.

I would come to learn that Alzheimer's disease is the result of abnormal protein build up in the brain. This leads to the progressive loss of brain cells. Symptoms usually start with short-term memory loss and an increasing inability to make rational connections soon follows. As the disease progresses, more and more memories and connections fall victim as dementia increases. Personalities of those affected can completely change. Hallucinations can occur if other forms of dementia develop. (As became the case with my mother, who later also developed Lewy body dementia). The line between physical reality and imagination often blurs. Eventually, bodily functions are lost, and the body "forgets" how to move. The ability to use the toilet, bathe, dress, and feed oneself deteriorate.

I did more research and learned that the disease gets its name from psychiatrist and neuropathologist Dr. Alois Alzheimer. He was the first doctor to publish a case of what he called "presenile disorder" in 1906. A colleague of his later dubbed it Alzheimer's disease. I often wonder how Dr. Alzheimer would feel about that. Because of what the disease does, his surname has now come to invoke dread in people and families around the world.

Most people think Alzheimer's just affects the memory, but it is ultimately fatal. As I once read somewhere, you probably know a cancer survivor. You do not know an Alzheimer's survivor and it is the way people die with Alzheimer's that can be the hardest to watch. No one dies from the disease itself—they die from its complications. As their minds dissolve away, so do their bodies. They forget how to chew and swallow, leading to massive weight loss. It can also lead to accidentally inhaling food, which results in aspiration pneumonia. At some point they usually become bedridden. This increases the chance of forming fatal blood clots. Or they contract infections that turn deadly to their weakened bodies.

Alzheimer's is such an awful word because there is no hope inside of it. As of this writing, it is the 6th leading cause of death in the United States. And yet, of the top 10 deadliest diseases, it is the only one with no effective treatment or cure. It comes with a 0% survival rate. Though there are at least a dozen theories, no one truly knows what causes it or how it works. The world of modern medicine has absolutely nothing hopeful to offer you after the word Alzheimer's. They can only say things like, "Get your affairs in order," and "Prepare for it to get worse over time."

I have been watching all this unfold for my mother over the past four years since her diagnosis. She now soils herself daily. She needs to be fed by hand because she's forgotten how to use utensils and doesn't recognize a plate of food. Her sentences rarely make sense. She is either angry or depressed much of the time. She no longer knows my name or grasps that I'm her daughter. She doesn't know anyone anymore. Her body is slowly shutting down. She has lost weight, and her already thin frame has grown more frail. Her body seems to have forgotten how to walk, and so she is either in bed or a chair all day. At her last doctor's appointment, we were given one year as an estimate of time left with her.

I have swum in a sea of emotions about her condition, especially in the beginning. Some days I can manage to tread through calmer waters. Other days it feels like I am drowning while a storm thrashes giant, salty waves over my head.

On those bad days, I suffer depths of pain I did not know were possible. I have suffocated myself with questions that seemed to have no answers. *Why Mom?* Could this have been prevented? How much time do we have left? How much worse will it get? How do I handle grieving her while she's still here?

So often I wanted to run away from it all, but something in me knew that I couldn't. Instead, I ran straight into it.

Four years after her diagnosis, my husband and I packed up our lives in Los Angeles and moved back to the tiny Idaho town where I grew up. I wanted to be there so I could help my father with Mom's increasing care needs. I decided to stare straight at this monster of a disease. I didn't know then I would see past all my questions and into a deep quiet where they no longer needed to be answered.

Yes, it has been hard. It has been ugly. It has been cruel. And... it has been the most profoundly transformative experience of my life. It has helped me understand the unequivocal power of Love. It has shown me where to find absolute peace.

This book is my attempt to share that with you. The word "Alzheimer's" may have no hope inside of it, but the experience of walking its journey does. If you find you must be forced to walk it as I have, I want you to have the gift of hope that others haven't offered. Underneath the disease is an ever-present opportunity to see the truths of life and Love.

I have found new levels of Grace and strength through this experience with my mom. I have written this book to share what I have seen with you. I wish for every human being going through a similar experience to have a piece of what I have found.

I hope that you will see more than my personal story in this small book. I want you to see what is behind the story. This book may seem like it's about me and my mom, but it's also about how we humans can see all life in a completely different way. It's to let you know that no matter what life looks or feels like, Love is untouchable and unchangeable. This book has five short chapters sharing the five biggest lessons I've learned from my mom. But really, they're all different versions of the same thing. Love is. Period. Seeing that is where we can always find hope, no matter how ugly the circumstances.

Love Doesn't Care If You Forget

"I haven't forgot... I just can't remember."

Winnie The Pooh

I had been preparing for the moment for over two years. Well, as much as one can prepare for such a thing. I tried to brace myself, to steel myself for it. I constantly reminded myself that the moment would come. Maybe if it doesn't catch me by surprise, I reasoned, it won't feel so sharp. I hoped by constantly reminding myself of its inevitability, it would somehow make it easier to handle. The voice in my head was on repeat.

"There will come a time when your mother doesn't know your name."

"There will come a day when your mother doesn't know who you are."

"There will come a moment when your mother will forget you." If I say it enough times, maybe it won't hurt so bad.

Despite my idea that these mantras would help, they didn't. The knowing still sat like a lead weight in the back of my mind since the day of her Alzheimer's diagnosis.

"Heartbreak is coming. It's coming and you can't stop it."

And come it did. But not at all as I had expected. I couldn't have known then that the gift of a broken heart is that it shows you where Love isn't. Love won't be found in the fragments of what was, and so you have to go looking for it elsewhere. The day my mother forgot me is the moment a different kind of journey began for us.

It happened over the Christmas holiday, two years after her diagnosis. Mom was wandering the house one night; a common byproduct of Alzheimer's dementia. She would often wake up anxious, confused, or scared. She would start looking for random things or just walk around the house, I assume trying to find a solution to the anxiety she felt, but couldn't understand. She came into the room my husband and I were sleeping in. I woke up as she was turning back out the door. I followed her to the living room and saw fear, nervousness, and sadness all over her face.

"What's wrong, Mama?" I asked.

She looked at me with confusion swimming in her eyes.

"This is my home," she said, "but I don't know who you people are." She was on the verge of tears.

This was it. It had begun—the forgetting of us. This would be the first time I had to face the fact that I, and others in her life, were slipping away. Her damaged mind was losing its ability to hang on to us.

This was the moment I had been dreading for years, and yet somehow, I felt no dread. The only way I know how to explain it is to say that I wasn't there. Instead, a sort of Grace took over and took my place. Brianne, who had worried endlessly about this moment, was gone. Brianne, who feared losing her mother, was not in attendance. Not an ounce of my awareness was thinking about me or my feelings. It didn't occur to me to consider myself, to recognize that this was a painful moment for me. I was focused entirely on the scared woman in front of me.

The Grace that took over spoke for me. "Oh, I see. That must be scary. Well, I can tell you we are all people who love you. We're all here, in your home, because we love you."

"You do?" she asked, and I watched the fear slip a little.

"Yes indeed. We love you a whole lot. That's why we're here," Grace reassured her.

I could see a sense of ease slip in through cracks, so I thought I would take a chance.

"Do you remember you have a daughter?" I asked.

"Yes," she said with hesitancy.

"Do you remember her name is Brianne?"

"Yes," she sounded a bit more sure.

"Well, that's me!" I said with the warmest smile I knew I'd ever smiled.

I watched the fear disappear from her eyes the way fog burns away from rays of the sun. Everything about her softened. She smiled the sweetest smile, and my mama reached out to me for the most amazing hug we had ever shared. Actually, it was more than a hug; it was the first time I knew what it meant to be embraced. We embraced each other. She pulled away, looked at me with the most loving eyes, then we embraced again. I don't think my mother and I have ever been wrapped in a moment filled with so much Love.

After a few moments, I asked if she was okay. A bit sheepish and unsure, she said yes, she thought so. My father had woken up at some point and joined us. He gently touched her shoulders and said he would take her back to bed. I saw a tiny bit of fear flash back in her eyes. I reassured her I would see her in the morning and the smile returned. "Alright, good night," she said.

I went back to my room and curled up next to my husband. Then Brianne returned, with all her fears, worries, and concerns. The tears and sobs flowed freely. My husband, knowing there were no words to say, just held me. I'm sure he felt horrible to see me hurting and unable to help. I didn't know how to convey to him that I was in deep pain, but also, that I was all right. I had seen something in that moment with my mom. I didn't have the words yet to describe the experience, but I knew it had been powerful. It had transformed the way I saw things. At first, I thought it changed the way I saw dementia. Years later though, the experience continues to permeate the way I see all of life.

I reflect back on this moment often. The first few times I tried to explain my experience it seemed that I wasn't accurately describing it. People thought that I was speaking to the power of Love, and its ability to "bring people back". They thought I found the moment beautiful because my mom remembered me. She remembered she had a daughter, and her daughter took away her fear and replaced it with Love, and all was well.

But that wasn't what was so powerful to me.

When my mother and I embraced, it wasn't as mother and daughter. It wasn't two people who had a shared history. There was no past or future in that moment. There was an absence of everything except the embrace. All ideas, all fears, all memories and expectations—none of it had any relevance in that moment. There was nothing remembered and nothing forgotten. There was only Love. There had only ever been Love, and Love would always remain. Everything else had been a series of dreams—some good, some bad. In that moment though, we were both fully awake.

And every single time I pause to think about it, to reflect on what happened between us, that knowing comes back. Perhaps not as clear, but powerful enough that it eases my fears and doubts. They begin to look like dreams.

I've had plenty of other moments with Mom when it seemed like Grace and Love were absent. Brianne and all her insecurities and fears have shown up and grieved deeply for the loss of her mother. Reminding Mom of who I am no longer "brings her back." She'll tell you she doesn't have a daughter and never did. But what I saw in that first moment, I saw so clearly that I know the possibility for Grace is ever-present. Dementia does not take that away from either of us.

I don't have to be afraid of Mom "losing her mind" because Love is not a concept or an idea. It cannot be lost when the mind loses the ability to hold thoughts. If thoughts go, if memories go, Love does not.

Love doesn't need your memory to exist.

Love doesn't care if you forget.

Love Doesn't Care How You Feel

"There is a secret medicine given only to those who hurt so hard they cannot hope."

Rumi

This morning, my mother looked at me with venom in her eyes. She yelled at me, told me to leave, said that she hated me, she didn't want me, and that she was going to kill me. She told me to go to hell, called me a bitch, and gave me a "fuck you" for good measure. All this because I was trying to help her out of bed. This is what she's like now when she's having a bad moment, consumed by feelings of anger.

It isn't the first time she's treated me, or others, this way. I'm guessing it won't be the last. This is the phase we're in. My poor, sweet mama is dealing with so much she can no longer understand—physically, mentally, or emotionally. It has to take a toll. I don't like her anger, at all, but I think I can understand it. And in the moments I can, her cruelty passes right through me. I have complete compassion and patience and can carry on loving her and caring for her with ease. In other moments though, it guts me. I have no idea what to do with it all, and I usually have to leave the room to regain my center. Sometimes I have a hard cry, like I did this morning after she flung those hate fueled words at me. I had to leave her for a moment and go into her bathroom to catch my tears and sob in my hands.

I'm okay with all these emotions though, mine and hers. It's a lot of feelings, but I'm no longer afraid of feelings. They don't mean what they used to mean to me. A few months after she had forgotten me for the first time, we had another experience that opened my eyes to something I had never noticed before.

I had been staying with my parents again, and one night I woke to the sound of my mom wandering through the house. My father was getting some much-deserved rest in another room, so I wanted to make sure she didn't wake him.

I had assumed I would find her upset, but I was not prepared for the state she was in. During her "normal" emotional episodes at that time, she would cry inconsolably and talk about things I couldn't understand. This night, however, her fear and panic were at levels I had never seen before. She wasn't scared or upset, she was utterly terrified. Not only did she not know where she was, but she had no idea who she was. She kept pulling at her clothes and touching her body and looking at her hands as if she had no idea why any of it was there. Through her sobs, she said over and over, "Who am I? I don't know who I am."

I had never seen someone in a state like that. She was totally disturbed and confused by her own existence. She acted as though she had been placed in an alien body, with no clue of how she got there and no memory of who she was before. She even looked physically different to me. She no longer looked like the mother I had known all my life or even the same person I had seen a few hours earlier. She was a vague replica of herself, as if her confusion was so great that even her facial features had forgotten how to form in their usual places and shapes.

It was horrible to see her that way, but again to my surprise, I did not cry or crumble. Instead, profound clarity broke through. I recognized with more certainty than I have ever felt in my life—I cannot fix this. This is too big. There is absolutely nothing in my power that can be done about this.

This revelation was not a devastating defeat; it was total freedom. I heard something loud and clear. "This is beyond you. You cannot make this okay. Making it okay is not your job. Life does not need you to fix this. Life just wants you here for this moment."

And so, my heart broke wide open for all the pain and fear that was pouring out of my mother. My heart opened up so wide that it swallowed her emotions whole. I bore witness to the experience she was lost in, but I did not get lost in it with her. I stood firm with my feet planted in clarity while Mom staggered in confusion. I waited until we both recognized we were in the same place.

I wiped her eyes for as long as she cried. I held her. I lay down with her in her bed and stroked her hair the way she did with me when I was little and scared. I was with her until the violent sobs slowed to softer whimpers—until the complete terror began to fade to simple distraction. Finally, she was worn out and the fear had subsided enough to allow her to close her eyes and sleep.

I watched over her all night long. I would occasionally drift off to sleep, but I would snap back awake at her slightest movement. I was afraid she would forget who I was or why I was there and the panic would start all over again.

While she slept, a sort of super-human feeling came over me. To see the resilience of your own heart in real-time is amazing. To recognize that this is something that could crush you, but see that it doesn't, opens new doors. To know the heart can expand so far that it can fit the infinite paradox of life and suffering inside of it gives you a glimpse into a new world. You begin to see there really is nothing to fear in this life. The human heart is not fragile at all; we just think it is.

Before this moment with my mother, I believed that my well-being was tied to hers. If she was having a good day, I could rest easy and enjoy the moment. But if she was upset, I had to share her pain. And that made sense. It seemed obvious that if you Love someone you should hurt along side them. It never occurred to me that Love doesn't have anything to do with those feelings.

As I watched my mother sleep, I thought more about her emotional states since the dementia had begun. She could go from upset and crying to happy and laughing in three seconds flat. When I thought about that, it made less sense to worry about how she was feeling in any given moment. What was the point of me being upset about her being upset when it was guaranteed to change?

The next morning, I saw this even more clearly. My mother got up and out of bed and had zero memory of the fear or disorientation. She was completely unfazed by the terror that had consumed her hours before. It was fascinating to see. There was no trace of the anxiety. None of those feelings had any more power over her. She could not recall prior thoughts and emotions and so she had no reason to worry about them. They left no lingering residue. She was free from anything she felt even moments before. It was the first time I began to understand that feelings can come and they can go, but they cannot do permanent damage. We have the capacity to feel deep and intense emotions and still be ok. And if that's true – we don't need to worry about how we're feeling in any given moment.

It was powerful for me to see that I could hold her pain without getting dragged into the fire with her. And also to see that she would be fine once the waves of her own emotions passed. Before this, I didn't know that we could be with those we Love as they struggle without losing ourselves. And I didn't know that we could be okay with our own pains if we don't hang on to them. I had spent most of my life either avoiding intense emotions, or trying entirely too hard to manage them. That night showed me how unnecessary that all is.

The gift of seeing that carried me through. That is how I could be hurt by her cruelty this morning, and also okay with it.

I knew it wouldn't last. I knew she would feel different at some point and so would I. So I let myself feel hurt. I let myself cry. I let her anger pierce my heart, because I knew my heart would be okay.

I have learned that we both get to have moments of intense feelings. We get to rage, and cry, and hurt, and curse the heavens. Because at some point we will "wake up", just like mom did on that morning, and the feelings will be gone. There's no need to worry about what's going to disappear anyway. I'm not afraid of these emotions or ashamed of them.

There are days when what is happening with my mother hits me in the gut. I will grieve on my knees until I can't breathe. I will shake my fists at the sky for the brutality of it all.

And in other moments, I am completely fine with being her emotional punching bag. I can stand strong and hold her while she yells or cries.

I don't try to do anything with any of it anymore. If I'm sad, I feel it. If I'm amused, I feel it. If I'm angry, I feel it. If I'm fine, I feel it. And the same goes for her. She gets to feel it all, too because none of this has anything to do with Love.

This is what it is to be alive. This is the package deal. We get to witness things coming into being, and going out of being. We get to relish in the things of life, but have to know that they cannot stay. Everything ends– bodies, minds, ideas, connections, personalities.

Of course, knowing this, seeing this, witnessing this over and over again every day—that comes with feelings. It comes with joys and sorrows, with pains and elations, with clarity and confusion. And all this is normal. It's all fine. Feelings are not problems. They just are. As humans, we feel.

We should not be afraid to feel, because Love is not in the feeling. It is the space that allows the feeling to happen. The more feeling, the bigger the space seems, and the larger Love looks.

Love wants you to feel, but it doesn't care how you feel.

Love Doesn't Care If You Understand

"Words are better off felt than understood."

-Sanober Khan

Mom started losing words as the dementia progressed. She's still pretty verbal for her late stage, but her vocabulary is limited. The word 'dog', for example, has become a placeholder for all kinds of things. She may say, "I want that dog," but actually mean she wants a drink or something else we can't decode.

Also, the words she has left don't arrange themselves in coherent sentences very often. She will still talk to you and engage in short conversation, but it has little meaning in the way you want it to.

And yet...Mom and I can still have great conversations. She will say something, and I will say something in return. And to watch us, it looks like we're carrying on and talking as anyone else would. People see us interact and ask, "What did she say?" My response is usually, "I have no idea." It's surprising how little that matters, though.

I've come to see that pretty much everything we say to each other is always a nonsensical version of the same thing.

"I'm here," she laughs and giggles.

"I know."

"I'm here," she cries and sobs.

"I know."

"I'm here," she curses and yells.

"I know."

Expressing and receiving. Stating and acknowledging. That's all she and I are ever really doing. And I find our gibbered conversations utterly beautiful—more and more so, the less she understands. We don't have to concern ourselves with getting it right. We don't have to carefully choose our words or worry about feeling awkward. There is so much freedom in being with someone and knowing that trying to understand each other is pointless. Now...we can simply be with each other.

This is why I began to Love being in the presence of my mother. Even when it's hard. Even when it sucks. Even when it crushes me. She's teaching me a different kind of Love. Something just beyond my intellectual understanding happens to me when I am with her. She is constantly pointing me toward the deepest secrets and treasures, asking me to open doors to worlds I otherwise would've never known.

Under the surface of all our experiences together, I keep hearing her beckoning me to keep looking. It is a call that I can't ignore or turn away from. Her voice whispers in my mind:

"I'm not in my words, you won't find me in what I say. Don't look for me there. I'm not in my past, you won't find me in our memories. Don't look for me there. I'm not in my actions, you won't find me in how I behave. Don't look for me there."

The disease has hidden her away, and she is nowhere to be found in the world I once knew. And so I have to go looking for her elsewhere. Like I'm on a scavenger hunt for my soul. It's a strange thing. The most difficult experience I have ever faced has become my awakening. I cannot wrap my mind around that. I don't know how to reconcile it. This thing that guts me to my core, is the same thing that has shown me more of life and Love than I knew possible. What do you do with that?

I'm beginning to see that the answer is: nothing.

We want to believe that life is supposed to make sense, but Mom has shown me that it doesn't. It is an infinite paradox that will never cohere the way we want. We actually miss out on much of life when we try to make sense of it. I'm learning that we only ever get to see and experience a tiny sliver of life, but we innocently make conclusions about the infinite whole based on the assumptions we've made about the tiniest part.

Ultimately, life will never actually make sense. We humans crave order and reason and cause and effect, and when we can't find them, we assume something is wrong. When really, life just does what it does, rarely with the kind of reason we would like. If you can broaden your gaze, you will find that there is space in life for these incompatibles; these absurdities. We may think certain things cannot co-exist, but that is just the limits of our own understanding, not any real truth.

In this existence, chaos and creation will always share the same space. So will beauty and ugliness, life and death, Love and grief, and confusion and clarity. None of this will ever make sense to the part of us that wants to understand.

I'm finding the less I try to make sense of it all—Mom, the disease, life and what's happening—the more sense it makes. I don't understand it, but I can live it.

It's a good thing Love doesn't care if I understand.

Love Isn't Personal

"We often confuse what we wish for with what is."

Neil Gaiman

Once upon a time in the land of my mother's mind, there was a space reserved for me, Brianne, her daughter. Things have changed. Where once there may have been my face, my name, dates and details tied to my existence– now there is an increasing emptiness. The space held for me is turning blank.

The fearful question I had for so long was: then what happens? If I disappear, where does the love go? If life smashes me to pieces, does love shatter with it? The answer I've seen is that it depends on what you think Love is.

I recently saw a friend ask people on social media to tell her what they thought love was. She received a wide array of answers. Many people thought love was some version of putting other people before yourself. Several people mentioned that love was a choice, it was actions, it was giving. A few acknowledged that the answer was hard to put into words.

I can't claim to have a perfect definition of Love. Over and over in this journey with my mom, though, life is showing me what Love isn't. And one thing is clear to me—Love is not personal. I'm seeing that most of what we think Love is, and where it resides, is nothing more than our personal ideas. *We think Love is what we want it to be.* But if that's true, what happens when life takes away those ideas? What if it cannot be anything like you wanted? What are you left with?

In my mother's world, she and I have no story or history together. I won't find Love in our past. She says she never had children, so I can't find Love in any of my ideas of what a mother/daughter relationship should be. To her, I'm not much of anything at all, no different than any other person. And she is no longer the woman I called Mom as a child. All the warm and comfortable things you might think of inside the word "mom" were taken from me. She is never going to cook my favorite meal again or call to see how I'm doing or soothe me when I'm hurting.

Life huffed and puffed and blew down every single home I thought Love lived in. No place of Love remained standing. I would search through the rubble and find nothing I could hold on to. That hurt, until I saw Love was never actually there in the first place.

I learned that Love is not housed in us, in our bodies or our minds. It is not contained in any of the things that change or disappear. I know this because my mother and I are fading away from each other and yet the Love is stronger than ever.

I have seen so much of my mother stripped away, and I don't

even exist in her world. Yet I am somehow left with more than what I had before. I feel more Love than ever. I've begun to wonder, what if Love is the absence of all our ideas? It looks to me like Love is what's left when everything else is gone. There is less and less of us, but more and more Love. So Love cannot be personal.

This first began to make sense to me when Mom's moods started to become more erratic. It was actually her anger that made it more obvious. As the dementia progressed, hatred and aggravation started showing themselves through her more and more often. These were brand new faces to me. They looked so foreign as they shaped my mother's facial features. When I was younger, I can remember her being upset sometimes, but never the complete loathing that can come from her now. When she gets angry, I genuinely believe she is trying to melt the skin from your bones with her eyes. She looks vicious.

I most often get this look when I'm trying to help her, particularly with bathing or changing. Often, as I try to undress and wash her, she calls me a bitch and tells me to fuck off. My mother hated the F-word when I was growing up. Now she uses language that I would never have guessed she even knew.

It definitely hurt the first few times she hurled her anger in my direction but it was understanding the impersonal nature of it that gave me the ability to let her words pass through me. I began to recognize that Brianne, daughter, doesn't exist in her world. So Brianne, daughter, does not need to be cut by her anger. She's just expressing her current state of being, nothing more. Yes, it's directed toward me, the person standing in front of her, but it doesn't have anything to do with me. She is just expressing a pure emotion. I can't blame her. I'd probably be pissed off too if all I knew was that someone I didn't know was trying to take my clothes off. Anger seems like a perfectly valid reaction. But it's never personal. It's not about me.

Seeing this allowed me to carry on even though she was angry and mean. It also helped that after the part she didn't like was over she would calm down. After a shower, we usually had lunch. We'd sit on the couch and have one of our nonsensical conversations. When she was calm, I could easily make her laugh. Often, we'd have a good giggle over something silly. Her laugh is magic, especially now. Often in these moments, her face would light up, she'd look at me, smile with joy and say, "Oh, I like you!"

And here's the sticky thing... for a while I would use those moments of affection for my respite. "Oh!", my heart would leap with joy. "She recognizes me! She still loves me. There it is, there is the evidence. Phew!" But you see, when you go looking for Love in places it doesn't exist, you'll eventually wind up empty-handed. Because those moments come less and less often. She doesn't calm down as much or as easily. She doesn't sit and talk with me for as long. It's become harder to make her laugh. She rarely says she likes me. I get fewer scraps of acknowledgment and less evidence of her Love for me.

And this weighed on me until it occurred to me one day that if her anger is not personal, neither is her affection. That, too, is simply her expressing a current mood toward the person sitting next to her. None of it has anything to do with me. It may seem like this would be a deflating thought, but it set my heart free. I don't exist, but it's so obvious to me that

Love still does. My experiences with Mom are richer and deeper now than any other time that I can recall. I saw that I could change, she could change, but Love can't.

Of course I want to hear her laugh with me, not yell at me. And even though I've seen wondrous things about life and Love because of this disease, plenty of times it still hurts like hell. There is grief and rage and shame and guilt. It feels incredibly personal in those moments. How dare life do this to my mom! How much pain am I going to have to endure? Why must this be so hard for my family? It often smacks me in the face. But none of these feelings indicate a lack of Love. It's just what happens when we turn Love into something personal.

Personal love will always let you down at some point. We rarely realize we've made Love personal, but that's what we do when we try to fit it inside our own ideas of what it's supposed to be, look like, or feel like. Life doesn't care about meeting us on our terms. It doesn't care what we want. Hurt will always find its way to us through the cracks of our conditions.

What remains after all the conditions are gone, that is universal Love. Beyond all ideas is where Love always lives. It's what allows you to Love someone who is gone. It's how you can be touched by the words of someone you've never met. It's what breathes your lungs on your hardest days. It's the ever-present sun that exists behind the darkest clouds.

I have not seen or experienced anything in life more powerful than this.

Love is not personal.

Love Doesn't Care What You know

"In the same way that you need to stop talking to hear what others are saying, you need to stop thinking in order to find what life is all about."

Alan Watts

Because of my mother, I'm a member of a few online support groups for people who have Loved Ones with Alzheimer's and dementia. There is a statement of helplessness that I see over and over again from people in these groups. It's expressed in many different ways, but the underlying statement is: "I don't know how to do this."

That despondent feeling stems from so many things that those of us with this disease in our lives have to face. How do you be with someone who no longer knows you? How do you answer the same questions over and over and over and over and over again as their minds become more jumbled? How do you handle their terror and panic and anger? How do you handle your own? How do you deal with them constantly soiling themselves? How do you bathe them once they hate bathing? How do you keep going when you're utterly exhausted? How do you not lose it when they turn into a different person? How do you deal with loneliness and isolation because it got too uncomfortable for other people and they stopped coming around? How do you grieve someone who is gone but still there? How do you watch someone you love slowly disappear and die? How do you look yourself in the mirror when you've wished for their death?

All these questions and more come into your life when you have a Loved One struggling like this. When you look at any of those questions head-on for the first time, the answer is always "I don't know." I've come to see though, that none of us actually know how to do the hard parts of life ahead of time. It turns out, that's not a problem.

When it comes to the most difficult aspects of life that we will face, none of us knows ahead of time how to get through. We don't know exactly what to do or say, how we will make it, how we will get it done. And yet...somehow, moment by moment, we do.

I have never felt more incompetent and inadequate than I feel on this journey with my mother. It's an unfamiliar feeling because before now I prided myself on my ability to get things done with confidence. I once took apart a broken lawnmower, fixed it and put it back together (even though I knew absolutely nothing about lawnmowers) just to prove I could. I spent 6 hours with one grossly tangled string of Christmas lights one year, determined to keep working until there was an orderly display of twinkling lights in my window.

But Mom's condition cannot be fixed and it cannot be untangled. I have remained entirely unprepared to do any of the things that I do for her now. It's been years of learning and adjusting and I still have no idea what I'm doing most of the time. That's not much of a problem, though. When I'm not thinking about my own inadequacy, I do quite well. It seems to me that the part of me that worries about it all will always be inherently inept at dealing with it. Thankfully, something other than worry always shows up. I've noticed I have an ability to fumble my way through the awkwardness with ease. I piece together steps and strategies. I gain new understandings and have new ideas. Or just as often, life completely takes care of things without my involvement.

I have countless examples of life showing me how to do things or doing them for me.

I didn't know how I was going to deal with my mother not knowing who I was and I couldn't have imagined what to do if I had known she would panic when she didn't know who she was. And yet, in those moments, I didn't have to think about any of it. I showed up and something else took over.

I thought it would be difficult to uproot my life in California and move back to Idaho to care for her and help my father. I had no idea how I would manage it, and yet it all just turned into a series of steps. None of them were particularly difficult. I transitioned smoothly into a new rhythm.

I had no training on how to feed your parent. No classes on adult bathing. No preparation for dealing with incontinence messes. But even without directions, I figured it all out.

Life showed me how to handle it all through trial and error, Grace and humor, Love and dignity.

I had so much stress and worry about moving Mom into a care facility. I wasn't sure how to talk to my father about it. I didn't know how our family would afford it or how to start the process. I was wary of how strangers would care for her and how she would handle the drastic change. When the time came though, life stepped up to offer all the help I needed. My brother helped me talk with Dad, and we all sat down to figure out the costs and payments. My wonderful husband graciously took over researching the facilities in our area. A relative, whom I was unaware worked for an elder law attorney, offered help and connections to work out details. When we toured the facility that wound up being Mom's new home, the staff were all kind and caring. When we moved Mom in, it went well and she adjusted as best she could.

Over and over again, through this experience with my mother, I have come to see a truth of life. If there is something we actually need but don't know how to get or do, one of two things will always happen. Either life will take care of it for us, or we'll figure it out (which is just another way life takes care of it for us). When I look at any aspect of my life, I have no evidence to the contrary. I have always figured out what to do, how to do it, how to move past it or get over it. Or, life somehow took the issue off my plate.

And that tells me that there is some other incomprehensible aspect of life that exists beyond our knowing that takes care of things for us.

I have no better word for that aspect of life than Love.

Love takes care of us. Love does not abandon us. It does not drop us off in any remote corner of life, dust its hands of us and say, "Alright, you're on your own now. You'll get no more help from me."

It can certainly look this way at times though, can't it? In our darkest hours, it can seem as though the world is a bitter and cold place. The mere mention of the word Love can seem an insult in those times, but as I've been doing my best to illustrate in this book, I don't believe this is evidence for lack of Love. It's what happens when we are confused and look for Love where it doesn't exist.

When we focus on the disease, all we can see is what can be lost. We see all the things that are going wrong, all the things we cannot fix. And there we find despair, heartbreak, confusion, helplessness. But Love is still present. Beyond all ideas, thoughts, feelings, words, language, or anything, Love itself is what carries us when we cannot carry ourselves.

We often don't see it or understand it, until we do. It mostly moves in the background of life and only reveals itself to us as a byproduct of its workings. It's the same unknowable knowing that coordinates nature which we only see evidence of through a budding flower. It operates with precise timing—which rarely lines up with our desired schedules. It is the animating force of life which keeps everything in existence evolving into its next iteration. And evolution, to us, sometimes looks messy, chaotic, and brutal. But always, it moves us forward, and when the dust settles, we can see that.

I cannot claim to know why we face pain, struggle or confusion in this life, I only know that we all will. I consider it a blessing that Mom has shown me something else about it all, though. She's shown me that if you can look past the pain, life will offer things to soften the sharp edges. It will show you how to get through. It will give you moments of respite as you travel the sometimes painful journey of life.

The part of us that worries about what to do and how to do it cannot help us, but help happens of itself. We have permission to stop trying to figure it out and let life take over. It doesn't matter if we don't know how. Love does the work.

Love doesn't care what you know.

Conclusion

"We're all just walking each other home."

Ram Dass

Seeing my mother through this illness, in whatever way I do that, has been the greatest privilege of my life. I also understand why others in similar difficult challenges would not see it that way for themselves. I understand why people shrink from things like this, why they get uncomfortable, try to avoid it, or rage against it.

Because it also fucking sucks.

Life can fill us up with the most intense experiences. Our feelings can begin to grind against the edges of who we think we are and what life is supposed to be. And when that happens, it usually hurts. It rubs us raw. It can feel like it's gripping us at the seams and trying to tear us apart. Who could blame anyone for hating that?

But...Mom has shown me that if you can sit with that discomfort and look straight at it, you can shed the ideas of what you think life is supposed to be and that is when you can see the power of life as it is. Life doesn't have to make sense, but it can always be fully lived. The pain doesn't have to tear us apart; instead, it can tear away what isn't pure Love.

I've said hundreds of times that I would change things for Mom if I could, but this is a story line of life that I have no say over. And so, I'm adjusting my character around it. I'm letting life mold me into something else. I'm allowing life to show me things that I don't think I could have seen without this crappy plot twist.

I believe that for many of us, the most beautiful version of our humanity is on the other side of pain. Maybe we can learn to hold life with strength and Grace from the safety of an easy existence, but it looks to me that those are the things pain sifts from us. The beauty comes from learning to be with pain, to sit with it, not to fight it, fix it, scorn it or abolish it.

If I could give the gift that has been given to me, it would be showing others that we are so much bigger than any experience—no matter how hard, no matter how painful, no matter how scary. The worst thing that can happen to you in this life is that you will experience intense emotions. But you are entirely equipped to feel those things.

When you see that, you are free. There is nothing in this life that can truly break you. And if you keep looking at life in the quieter moments, when your own objections to it subside, that is when a deeper beauty reveals itself.

It's not that you live a fearless life or a painless life. It's that you shake hands with fear and pain when they come to your door. You look them in the eye with powerful confidence in your soul. You know that while they may enter your house, it is not within their power to tear the foundation. They can rip the wallpaper, break the glass, flip the furniture—but the structure will always remain sound. And life will make all necessary repairs.

I am grateful for being able to see something so profound in this journey with Mom, but I'm also still bitter about it. And I'm okay with that. I've learned to live comfortably inside this paradox because life will never stop being one. To try to untangle the beautiful from the ugly is painful and exhausting because it's an impossible task. They are both woven into the fabric of life. When you can see the full tapestry, it doesn't matter what the individual threads look like.

My mother no longer knows who I am, and I no longer get to have who she was. But where I can always find her, every single time without fail, is in the deepest places of Love. In all the ways in which Love truly exists - beyond words, beyond memories, beyond hopes and dreams. Love is the foundation. It is where we begin and where we end.

Yes, I hate the disease. I hate how it's changed her. I hate that we've all had to adjust so much. But in the quiet space beyond my own objections, I can see that those changes are still only on the surface. Underneath all the madness, infinite Love is still always available. And she was the one who taught this to me. This is a lesson I will never forget.

But even if I do, Love will not care.

Acknowledgments

My father may not be mentioned much in these pages, but I cannot possibly end this book without giving him the important acknowledgment that he deserves. He is the backbone of our family. He took on far more than I on this journey of caring for Mom and I am forever grateful. "Thank you" and "I Love you" are words that will never be able to hold the weight of their meaning here, but words are what I have. Thank you, Dad. I Love you.

Of course, Mom...You will never get to read or understand these words—but I hope that somehow you know you are helping people. Not just me, but those who have heard me share our story and been touched. Your legacy is Love, Mama. Thank you for letting me be part of it.

And my amazing husband. I don't know how I would have done any of this without you. Your support, your Love, your willingness to adjust, your understanding, your patience, your handling of the hard parts, your everything. Thank you, my Love. Thank you.

A deep thank you goes to Michael Neill, a man I call mentor. While this journey with my mother has been my greatest teacher, your shared wisdom is what allowed me to keep looking when all I wanted to do was close my eyes. I can't possibly know what this journey would have been like without your guidance. But I do know that your constant pointing in the direction of Love is one of the things life gave me to soften the sharp parts.

Much gratitude goes to Alexandra Franzen and Lindsey Smith who helped me see that a "tiny book" is just as valid as 300 pages. People are reading these words because you helped me complete just one small book, one small part at a time. Without you, I would still be trying to finish chapter one of a book that the world would never see.

About Brianne Grebil

Brianne is a writer, coach and teacher who has worked with people all over the world to help them see the powerful beauty and simple truths of life. She has written for Medium, Mind Body Green, and Love What Matters.

You can read all of Brianne's other work by following along on her website or social media accounts.

www.briannegrebil.com
Facebook: *briannegrebil*
Instagram: *briannegrebil*

Brianne has also created a website and social media accounts where you can share your own story of the journey through dementia, or read stories from others. You can find these stories, as well as other resources for Alzheimer's and dementia at Love and Dementia.

www.loveanddementia.com
Facebook: *loveanddementia*
Instagram: *loveanddementa*

If you enjoyed this book, consider writing a review on Amazon or sharing with your friends and colleagues.

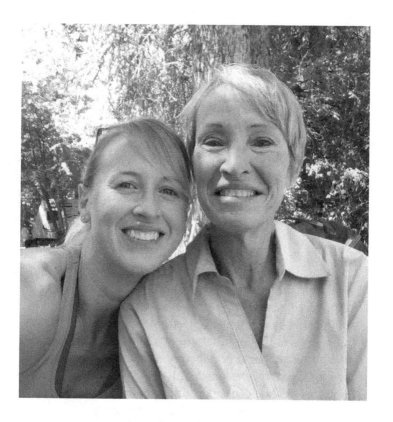

The author and her mother